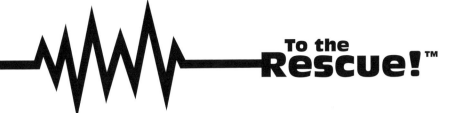

Ambulances
Ambulancias

Joanne Randolph

Traducción al español:
Eduardo Alamán

PowerKiDS press. & **Editorial Buenas Letras**™

New York

For Riley, Deming, and Hannah

Published in 2008 by The Rosen Publishing Group, Inc.
29 East 21st Street, New York, NY 10010

First Edition

Book Design: Greg Tucker
Photo Researcher: Nicole Pristash

Photo Credits: Cover, pp. 7, 11, 13, 15, 19, 21, 24 (top left), 24 (bottom left), 24 (bottom right) Shutterstock.com; p. 5 © www.iStockphoto.com/Hazlan Abdul Hakim; p. 9 © www.iStockphoto.com/Nancy Louie; p. 17, 24 (top right) © www.iStockphoto.com/David Dea; p. 23 © www.iStockphoto.com/Tana Minnick.

Cataloging Data

Randolph, Joanne.
  Ambulances–Ambulancias / Joanne Randolph; traducción al español: Eduardo Alamán.— 1st ed.
     p. cm. — (To the rescue!–¡Al rescate!)
  Includes index.
  ISBN 978-1-4042-7670-3 (library binding)
  1. Ambulances—Juvenile literature. 2. Emergency medicine—Juvenile literature. 3. Spanish language materials I. Title.

Manufactured in the United States of America

Websites: Due to the changing nature of Internet links, PowerKids Press and Editorial Buenas Letras have developed an online list of Web sites related to the subject of this book. This site is updated regularly. Please use this link to access the list: www.powerkidslinks.com/ttr/ambul/

Contents/Contenido

Ambulances save people's lives every day.

Las ambulancias salvan vidas todos los días.

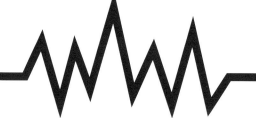

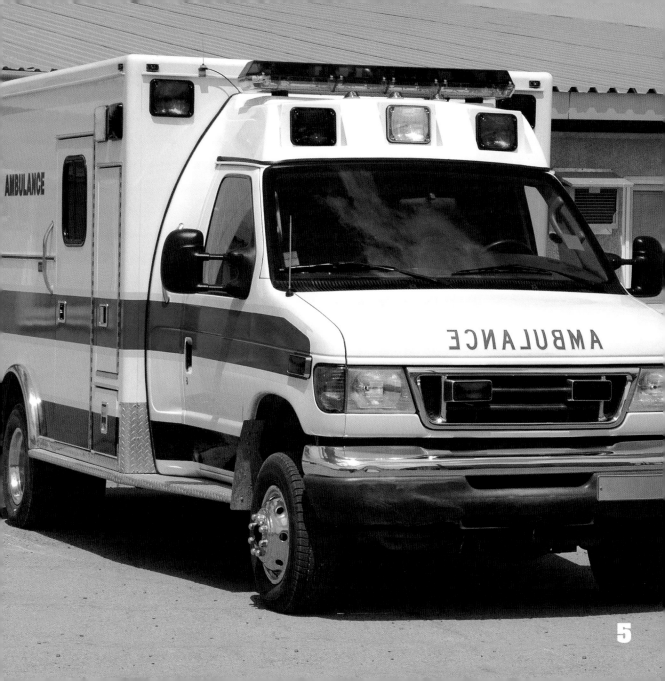

The people who drive ambulances are called EMTs or **paramedics**.

A quienes trabajan en las ambulancias se les conoce como EMT, que quiere decir técnicos en emergencias médicas. También se les llama **paramédicos**.

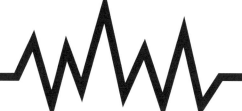

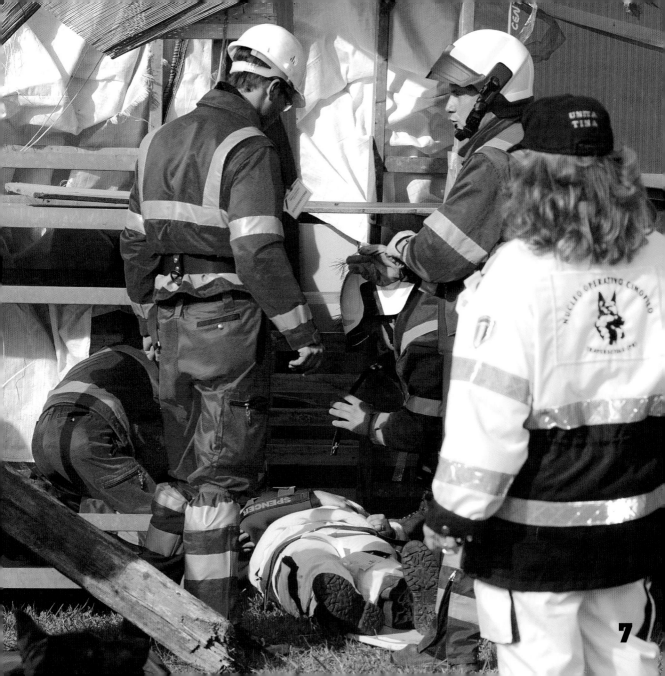

EMTs and paramedics help people who are sick or hurt.

Los EMT y los paramédicos ayudan a los heridos o a los enfermos.

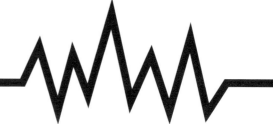

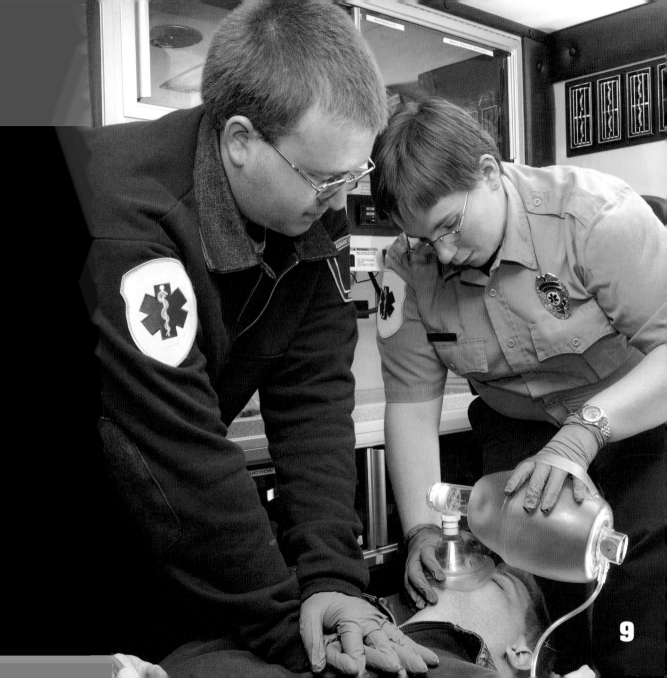

Ambulances have lights on top. The lights are turned on when an ambulance is on its way to help someone.

Las ambulancias tienen luces en el techo. Las ambulancias encienden estas luces cuando van a ayudar a alguna persona.

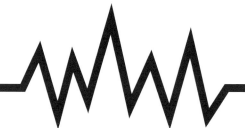

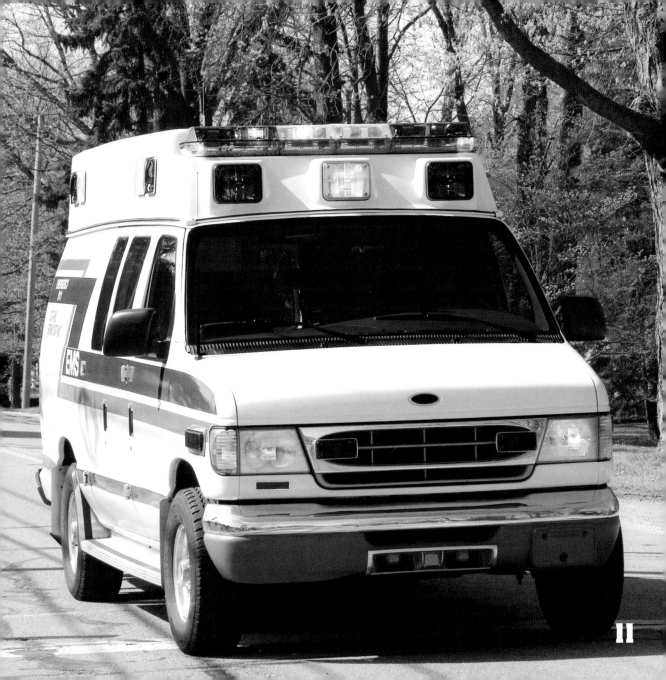

Sick people are put on a **stretcher** to ride in the back of the ambulance.

A los heridos los ponen en una **camilla** antes de subirlos a la ambulancia.

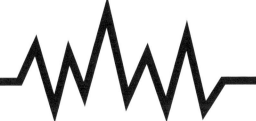

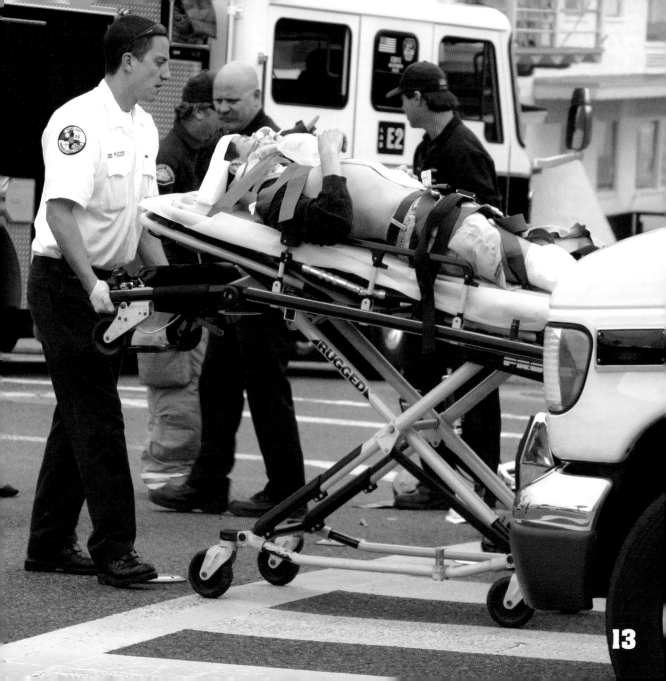

This is the inside of an ambulance. It has everything EMTs and paramedics need to do their job.

Esta es una ambulancia por dentro. Tiene todo lo que los EMT y los paramédicos necesitan en su trabajo.

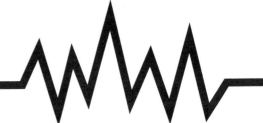

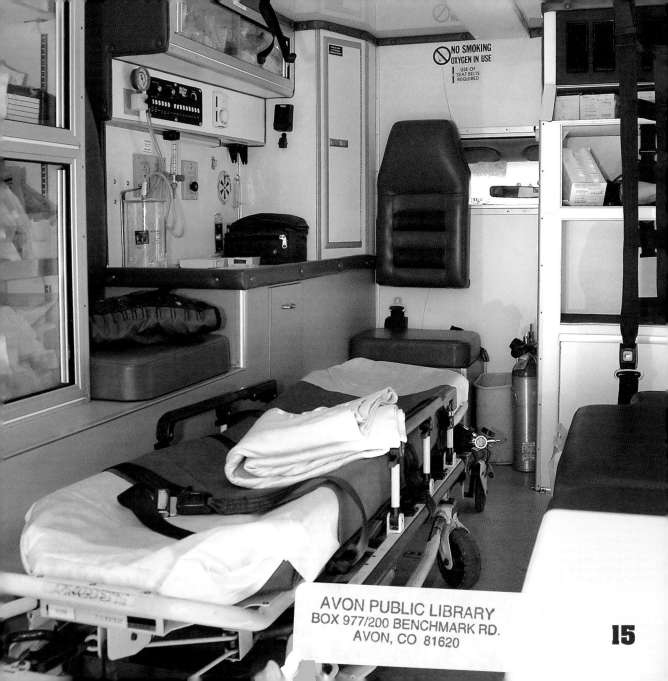

NO SMOKING
OXYGEN IN USE

USE OF
SEAT BELTS
REQUIRED

15

Ambulances bring people to the **hospital**.

Las ambulancias llevan a las personas al **hospital**.

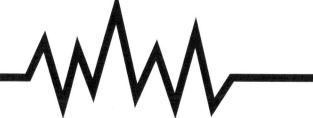

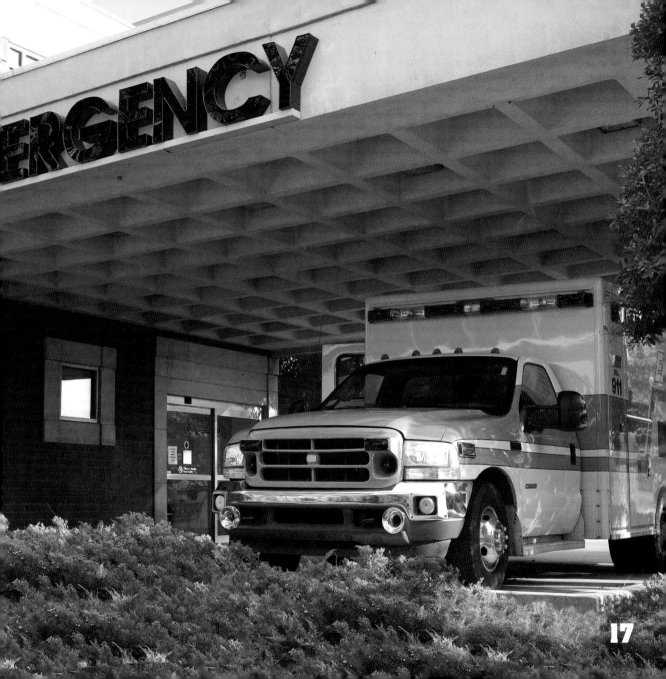

Ambulances are called to help out after a **car crash**.

Las ambulancias ayudan en los **accidentes de tránsito**.

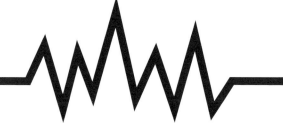

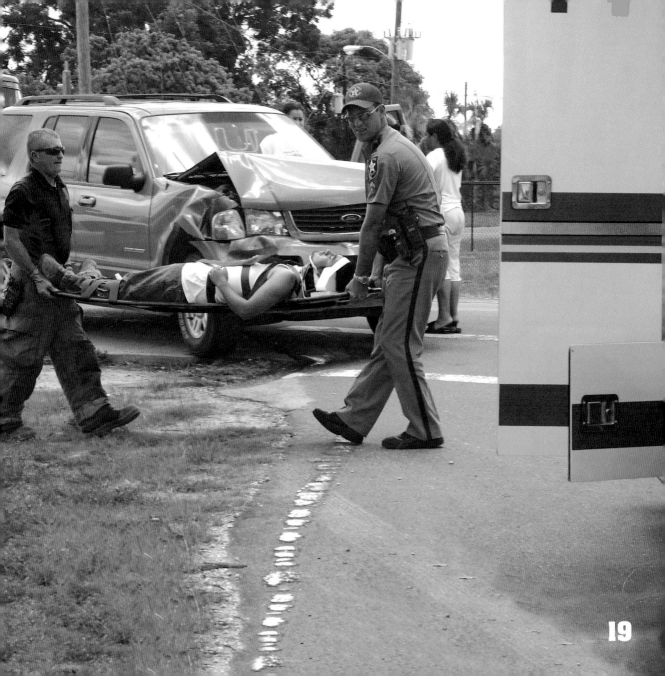

Ambulances help out anywhere someone could be hurt or sick.

Las ambulancias ayudan en todas partes a cualquiera que esté enfermo o lastimado.

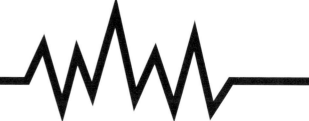

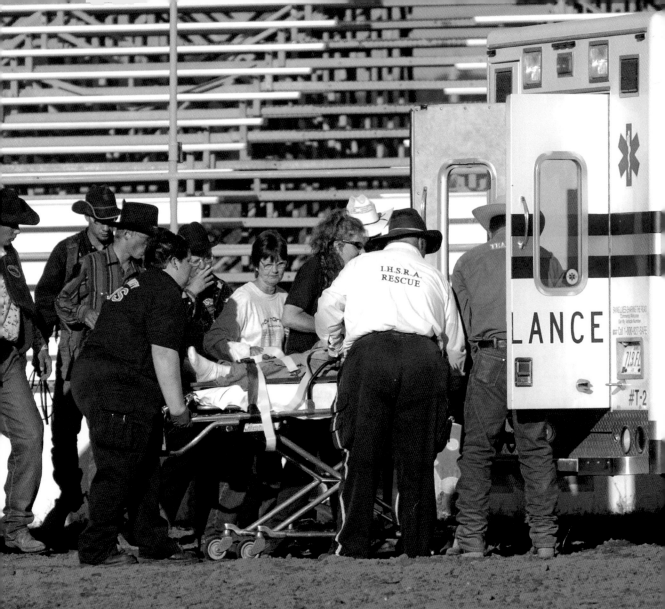

Thank goodness there are ambulances ready to help people in need!

¡Qué suerte tenemos de que las ambulancias siempre estén listas para ayudar a quienes lo necesiten!

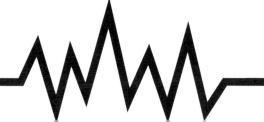

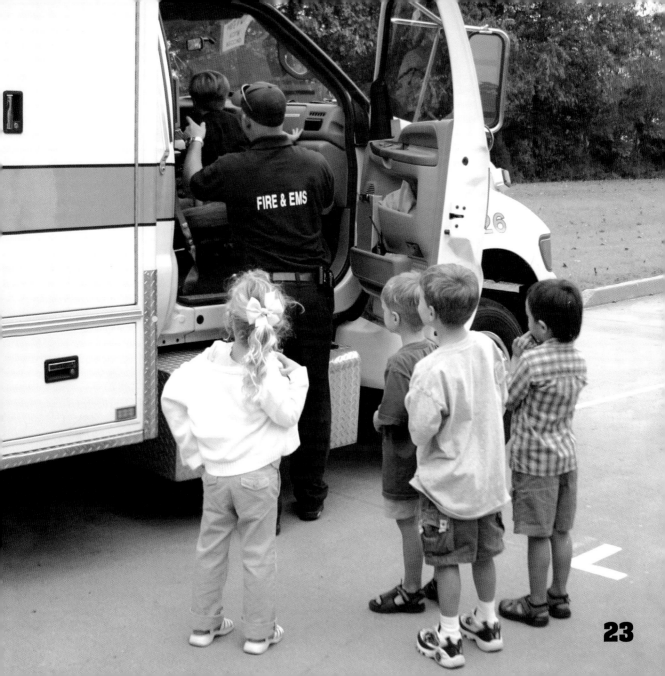

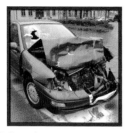

car crash / (los) accidentes de tránsito

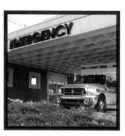

hospital / (el) hospital

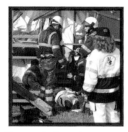

paramedics / (los) paramédicos

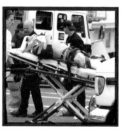

stretcher / (la) camilla

Index / Índice